Samson Chisele
Groesbeck Parham
Mulindi Mwanahamuntu

Histologic Outcomes for Cryotherapy-Ineligible Cervical Lesions

Samson Chisele
Groesbeck Parham
Mulindi Mwanahamuntu

Histologic Outcomes for Cryotherapy-Ineligible Cervical Lesions

LAP LAMBERT Academic Publishing

Impressum / Imprint

Bibliografische Information der Deutschen Nationalbibliothek: Die Deutsche Nationalbibliothek verzeichnet diese Publikation in der Deutschen Nationalbibliografie; detaillierte bibliografische Daten sind im Internet über http://dnb.d-nb.de abrufbar.

Alle in diesem Buch genannten Marken und Produktnamen unterliegen warenzeichen-, marken- oder patentrechtlichem Schutz bzw. sind Warenzeichen oder eingetragene Warenzeichen der jeweiligen Inhaber. Die Wiedergabe von Marken, Produktnamen, Gebrauchsnamen, Handelsnamen, Warenbezeichnungen u.s.w. in diesem Werk berechtigt auch ohne besondere Kennzeichnung nicht zu der Annahme, dass solche Namen im Sinne der Warenzeichen- und Markenschutzgesetzgebung als frei zu betrachten wären und daher von jedermann benutzt werden dürften.

Bibliographic information published by the Deutsche Nationalbibliothek: The Deutsche Nationalbibliothek lists this publication in the Deutsche Nationalbibliografie; detailed bibliographic data are available in the Internet at http://dnb.d-nb.de.

Any brand names and product names mentioned in this book are subject to trademark, brand or patent protection and are trademarks or registered trademarks of their respective holders. The use of brand names, product names, common names, trade names, product descriptions etc. even without a particular marking in this work is in no way to be construed to mean that such names may be regarded as unrestricted in respect of trademark and brand protection legislation and could thus be used by anyone.

Coverbild / Cover image: www.ingimage.com

Verlag / Publisher:
LAP LAMBERT Academic Publishing
ist ein Imprint der / is a trademark of
OmniScriptum GmbH & Co. KG
Heinrich-Böcking-Str. 6-8, 66121 Saarbrücken, Deutschland / Germany
Email: info@lap-publishing.com

Herstellung: siehe letzte Seite /
Printed at: see last page
ISBN: 978-3-659-69268-0

Zugl. / Approved by: Lusaka, University Of Zambia, Diss.,2010

HISTOPATHOLOGIC OUTCOMES OF CRYOTHERAPY-INELIGIBLE LESIONS

By DR. SAMSON CHISELE

DEDICATION

To the memory of my late father Mr. Mumba Blackson Chisele (Snr).

ACKNOWLEDGEMENT

I wish to thank the following people for their various contributions to this study:

Prof. Groesbeck Parham- Co Director, Cervical Cancer Prevention Program in Zambia, for the original concept and guidance throughout the study.

Dr. Benjamin Chi - Training Director, Centre for Infectious Disease Research in Zambia for all the technical support.

Dr.Gricellia Mkumba – Senior Consultant Obstetrician and Gynaecologist, University Teaching Hospital, for evaluating some of the study participants.

The University of Alabama at Birmingham's Centre of Infectious Disease Research in Zambia for partially funding this study, through a grant from the U.S. National Institutes of Health's Fogarty International Clinical Research Centre.

Kristin Elizabeth King and Jennifer Hallock for being part of the original study concept.

Mr Johnny Banda for analyzing the data.

Dr. Yusuf Ahmed - for editing the dissertation.

Finally, I am indebted to Dr. Mulindi Mwanahamuntu - Consultant Obstetrician and Gynaecologist, University Teaching Hospital and Co-Director of the Cervical Cancer Prevention Program in Zambia, for his relentless supervision.

ABSTRACT

Objectives To determine the association between high grade cervical intraepithelial neoplasia (CIN 2+) and individual acetowhite cryotherapy-ineligible lesion types, as determined by cervicography.

Design: a cross sectional study

Setting: Gynecologic Cancer Prevention Unit of the University Teaching Hospital, Zambia.

Population: Women referred to the study site for histologic evaluation of cryotherapy-ineligible lesions of the cervix were included in the study. Individual acetowhite lesion types which do not meet criteria for cryotherapy include those that (1) cover more than 75% of the transformation zone, (2) disappear into the endocervical canal, (3) contain abnormal vasculature (mosaicism, punctuations, or atypical blood vessels), and (4) are thick.

Main outcome measures: Histologic diagnosis of high grade cervical intraepithelial neoplasia (CIN 2+) for each cryotherapy-ineligible acetowhite lesion type of the cervix.

Results: A total of 130 women were enrolled into the study. After multivariable adjustment, there remained a significant association between lesions covering greater than 75% of the transformation zone and CIN 2+, OR 2.2 (95% CI 1.4-3.4). However, other individual cryotherapy-ineligible acetowhite lesion types were no longer associated with CIN 2+.

Conclusions: Cryotherapy-ineligible acetowhite lesions occupying greater than 75% of the transformation zone diagnosed on cervicography are associated with histopathologic outcome of high grade cervical intraepithelial neoplasia.

TABLE OF CONTENTS

TABLES

LIST OF ABBREVIATIONS

AIDS – Acquired Immune Deficiency Syndrome

CIN – Cervical Intraepithelial Neoplasia

HIV – Human Immunodeficiency Virus

HPV- Human Papilloma virus

HSIL – High Grade Squamous Intraepithelial Lesion

LEEP – Loop Electrosurgical Excision Procedure

LSIL – Low Grade Squamous Intraepithelial Lesion

UTH- University Teaching Hospital

VIA – Visual Inspection with Acetic acid

WHO-World Health Organisation

1.1. Background

Over the past decade, visual inspection of the cervix following application of dilute (3-5%) acetic acid (VIA) has been used together with adjunct digital cervicography as a promising alternative to the Papaniculou smear (Pap smear), in the screening of cervical cancer in resource-poor settings. VIA has a greater sensitivity than that of the Pap smear, and it is cost-effective, easy to learn, simple, safe, efficacious, acceptable, real-time in nature and easily adaptable for use in developing countries.[i, ii, iii] VIA has recently been shown to significantly reduce the incidence of cervical intraepithelial neoplasia (CIN) and cervical cancer as well as the mortality rates of the latter in developing country settings.[iv, v]

According to the World Health Organisation (WHO) and the International Agency for Research on Cancer (IARC) [14] a woman is said to be VIA positive if after application of acetic acid to the uterine cervix, there is detection of distinct, well-defined acetowhite areas with sharp borders that are close to the transformation zone. In "see and treat" programs involving the use of immediate cryotherapy for positive tests, criteria have been established to triage lesions that can be treated with cryotherapy and those that are cryotherapy-ineligible and thus require histologic evaluation or treatment with loop electrosurgical excision procedure (LEEP). Those criteria are as follows: acetowhite lesions covering more than 75% of the transformation zone, lesions disappearing into the endocervix beyond complete visualization, lesions showing abnormal vessels (mosaicism, punctuations, and atypical vessels) or thick lesions.[vi] These criteria are believed to represent high grade cervical disease.[vii]

Cryotherapy and LEEP are two safe, effective, relatively simple and inexpensive outpatient methods used for the treatment of pre-cancer of the cervix. The major practical differences between the two methods are that LEEP involves excision of the tissue and hence provides a tissue specimen that allows for histologic verification of the diagnosis, LEEP equipment is considerably more expensive, and LEEP requires more training to use safely. On the other hand, cryotherapy is an ablative method that involves destroying the tissue and thereby leaves no sample for histology, but it can be safely conducted by non-specialist providers including nurses with proper training. Meta-analysis of randomized clinical trials that evaluated the comparative effectiveness of cryotherapy with therapies such as LEEP, conization and laser, have concluded that the above treatments are equally effective in controlling CIN.[viii, ix]

From the foregoing comparisons and contrasts, the most practical and cost-effective method of treatment of CIN in low-resource settings is cryotherapy, provided the lesion is wholly ectocervical in location. LEEP is the treatment of choice if the lesion involves the endocervical canal.

1.2. Statement of the problem

Despite its many advantages, VIA has some draw backs that need to be investigated. The major problem is its low specificity. The incidence of negative and low-grade cervical disease outcomes when VIA positive lesions are histologically evaluated has been shown to be high. It ranges from 8.2 to 61.1 % for any dysplasia and 9.8 to 63.4 % for high grade cervical lesions.[x,xi,xii]

In the Cervical Cancer Prevention Program in Zambia, over 60.8% of women diagnosed with high grade cervical disease on VIA end up with negative or low-grade cervical disease when evaluated by histopathology. This means

9

approximately two thirds of women undergo LEEP to obtain histopathologic evaluation when they do not need it. This problem has been perpetuated by existing criteria that triages cervical lesions with certain VIA based morphologic criteria for histologic evaluation on grounds that the lesions may represent early cervical cancer.

1.3. Study justification

There is a paucity of published information on the correlation between specific digital cervicographic findings and histopathologic outcomes. Most published studies [11, 12] have evaluated the final histologic outcome of cervigrams in general but have not addressed histologic outcomes of individual surface morphologic criteria as determined by cervicography. As a result, evidence based explanations for false positive VIA lesions are still lacking. This study proposes to provide some of this evidence by isolating particular digital cervicographic criteria that correlate well with histologic diagnosis of high-grade cervical disease.

Information gathered from this study will be important in evaluating the accuracy of criteria used for performing histologic evaluation of acetowhite lesions of the cervix. Further, this information will be useful in helping reduce the over-treatment linked to the current criteria for histologic evaluation of acetowhite lesions of the cervix.

2.0. LITERATURE REVIEW

Cervical cancer is the most common cancer among women in developing countries. According to World Health Organization projections, in 2005 there were over 500,000 new cases of cervical cancer and 275,000 deaths. Over 90% of deaths occurred in developing countries including sub-Saharan Africa.[xiii] Zambia has the sixth highest incidence of cervical cancer in the world and the second highest in Africa, at 61.1 per 100,000 women.[xiv]

Various epidemiological studies have identified a number of risk factors that contribute to the development of cervical cancer precursors and cervical cancer. Key among these factors is persistent infection with certain oncogenic types of human papilloma viruses (HPV).[xv, xvi] About 80% of young women who become infected with HPV have transient infections that clear up within 12-18 months. [xvii,xviii] It appears that it takes about 10 to 20 years for progression of cervical precursors to invasive cancer. However, in HIV-infected women, CIN of any grade is more prevalent,[xix, xx] has a higher incidence,[xxi,xxii] progresses more rapidly[xxiii] and is diagnosed at a higher grade than in HIV-uninfected women.[xxiv] The strength of these associations increases with the degree of immunosuppression.[xxv] This is exemplified by the fact that HIV-infected women suffering from the severest forms of immunosuppression (CD4+ count <200/μL) seem to be at greatest risk for developing high grade CIN.[xxvi, xxvii]

Various studies have demonstrated that cervicography improves detection of cervical disease. Ferris et al (1993)[xxviii] evaluated the use of cervicography as an adjunct to cytology screening. In this study, they concluded that cervicography detected twice the number of patients with premalignant disease as the Pap smear alone, and correctly identified invasive cancer which was missed by Pap smear. In a study to evaluate the feasibility of screening by cervicography, Cecchini et al

(1993)[xxix] concluded that cervicoscopy was poorly specific but increased the detection rate of CIN 2-3 at relatively low cost. Frisch et al (1994)[xxx] assessed the predictive value of VIA as an adjunct to Pap smear. It was shown in this study that VIA significantly improved the predictive value of negative cytologic screening results. Denny et al (2002)[xxxi] investigated the influence of concurrent sexually transmitted infections on the test characteristics of VIA in a South African study and found that there were no significant differences in the sensitivity and specificity of VIA relating to the presence or absence of *N. gonorrhea*, *C. trachomatis* or *T. vaginalis*. The specificity of VIA was, however, significantly lower among human immunodeficiency virus (HIV)-positive women.

However, other studies have questioned the reliability of cervicography as a screening tool for cervical cancer. Baldauf et al (1997)[xxxii] compared the reliability of cytology with that of cervicography when screening for neoplasia of the cervix and analyzed the causes of false positive and false negative results with both methods. The results of cytology and cervicography were correlated with colpohistologic findings. Whatever the clinical criteria (patient's age, parity, pregnancy or history of cervical treatment), the rate of false positives with cervicography was always higher than with cytology, as was the rate of false negatives, except in pregnant women. The study concluded that cervicography does not seem to offer a worthwhile alternative to cytology for cervical screening.

Data is scanty on the histologic outcomes of acetowhite lesions based on specific morphologic criteria. However, various studies have been done to show that Pap smear based diagnosis of high grade squamous intraepithelial lesions (HSIL) correlate well with histologically proven high grade cervical disease. Similar methodologies can be applied to study histological outcomes in the see and treat protocol for patients with certain VIA morphologic criteria.

Numnum et al (2005)[xxxiii] evaluated the incidence of CIN 2 and CIN 3 in patients with an high grade squamous intraepithelial lesions (HSIL) Pap smear using a see-and-treat protocol. Women referred from local health departments to a university-based colposcopy clinic for evaluation of an HSIL Pap smear result were evaluated for inclusion in a see and treat protocol. All eligible patients underwent colposcopy to rule out an obvious cervical carcinoma followed by an immediate LEEP to remove the transformation zone. Specimens were analyzed for the presence of CIN and the incidence of CIN 2 and CIN 3 was determined. Of the 51 LEEP specimens available at the time of publication, 4 of 51 had no evidence of CIN (8%), 4 of 51 (8%) had CIN 1, 18 of 51 (35%) had CIN 2, and 25 of 51 (49%) had CIN 3. Eighty-four percent of patients had either CIN 2 or CIN 3, resulting in an over treatment rate (CIN 1 or less) of 16%. The study concluded that the use of a see and treat protocol for patients with an HSIL Pap smear result may be an acceptable treatment option because of a high incidence of CIN 2 and CIN 3.

Szurkus et al (2003)[xxxiv] retrospectively reviewed all patients who underwent LEEP for HGSIL on Pap smear. None of the patients evaluated had prior cervical biopsies. Histologic results were also correlated with visual (colposcopic) findings at the time of LEEP. Of 104 patients undergoing LEEP, 63 (61%) had pathologic evidence of cervical intraepithelial neoplasia (CIN) grade 2 or greater. Of the 63 patients with ≥CIN 2, 34 (54%) had a normal or low-grade colposcopic findings, indicative of the poor correlation between visual and histologic findings. They conclude that despite lack of correlation between colposcopic and histologic results, HGSIL on Pap smear is an appropriate indication for LEEP.

13

Charoenkwan et al (2006)[xxxv] studied the final histopathologic outcome of 48 women with squamous cell carcinoma (SCC) on cytology. The medical records and computerized colposcopic database of patients with SCC on cytology were reviewed. While 31 (64.6%) of the 48 patients with SCC on cytology had a final pathologic diagnosis of high-grade squamous intraepithelial lesions (HGSIL), only 16 (33.3%) actually had invasive cancer.

Using a predictive model to reduce the number of negative specimens following histologic evaluation has also been studied. Howells et al (2000) [xxxvi] used a retrospective review of patient notes and audit database to analyse biopsies of large loop excision of the transformation zone of the cervix to identify factors associated with negative histology; and to develop predictive models in order to reduce the number of negative loop excisions. They concluded that using a predictive model can reduce the number of negative LEEP specimens, but at the expense of continued cytological and colposcopic surveillance and cannot be recommended in normal practice.

The conclusion in Howell's study is well placed in high resource settings with good colposcopic and cytologic facilities and high patient compliance. However in low resource settings that use a single visit VIA based see and treat protocol, there would be no need for continued surveillance of patients in the predictive model considering that all women with abnormal acetowhite lesions will receive treatment in form of cryotherapy or LEEP.

2.1. Eligibility Criteria for Cryotherapy

For a VIA positive acetowhite lesion to be eligible for cryotherapy the following conditions should be satisfied:

14

1. the lesion should occupy less than 75% of the transformation zone –Large or extensive high grade lesions involving more than three quadrants of the cervix should be investigated for the possibility of early invasive cancer.[xxxvii]

2. the lesion should not extend into the cervix beyond complete visualization – Lesions disappearing into the endocervix have been known to be resistant to cryotherapy mainly because their full extent can not be ascertained and therefore the minimum temperature of -20° Celsius which is required for cryonecrosis to occur can not be guaranteed at the distal or cranial limit of this type of lesion.[xxxviii]

3. there should be no abnormal vessels(such as punctations, mosaicism and atypical vessels) or bleeding. As the neoplastic process closely approaches the stage of invasive cancer, the blood vessels can take on increasingly irregular, bizarre patterns. Appearance of irregular vessels often indicates the first sign of invasion.[xxxix] Therefore lesions with abnormal vessels should be investigated for early cancer.

4. The lesion must not be thick. Early preclinical cancer may appear as dense, thick, chalky white areas with surface irregularity and nodularity and with raised and rolled out margins.[39] Such lesions may not present with abnormal blood vessels and may not bleed on touch. If cryotherapy is performed on such lesions a biopsy must be taken before hand to exclude early cancer, otherwise LEEP is preferable.

5. The lesion must be adequately covered by the largest available cryotherapy probe or the lesion extends less than 2mm beyond the edge of the cryotherapy probe. Adequate freezing is achieved when the margin of the ice ball extends 4-5mm past the outer edge of the cryotip. Therefore a lesion that is within 2 mm

away from the outer edge of the cryotip will be adequately covered by the ice ball. A satellite lesion is one that is distant from the squamo-columnar junction.[xl]

3.0. STUDY DEFINITIONS

3.1. Digital Cervicography

Digital cervicography involves obtaining and evaluating a photographic image of the cervix using a digital camera fixed with a magnifying lens. This photograph, also called a cervigram, can be used, among other things, for education of patients, distance tele-consultation for indeterminate results and for continuing education of providers.

3.2. Cryotherapy

This is an ablative mode of treating pre cancer lesions of the cervix by freezing the affected part of the cervical epithelium, thereby killing the pre cancer cells. This is achieved by placing a cryotherapy probe in contact with the cervix. The probe is then frozen by a refrigerant gas (mainly compressed nitrous oxide or carbon dioxide) and a ball of ice forms around it, cooling the cervix to temperatures below -20degrees for at least one minute. This process causes cryonecrosis of cervical epithelium.

3.3. Cryotherapy Ineligible Lesions

These are by default, lesions that do not meet criteria for cryotherapy. They include: acetowhite lesions that extend into endocervix beyond complete visualization; lesions occupying greater than 75% of the transformation zone; lesions with abnormal vessels (mosaicism, punctations or atypical vessels), thick lesions and satellite lesions.

16

3.4. High Grade Cervical Disease

In this study, high grade cervical disease refers to histopathologic findings of moderate (CIN 2) or severe (CIN 3) cervical intraepithelial neoplasia, or invasive carcinoma.

3.5. LEEP

Loop electrosurgical excision procedure (LEEP) is a mode of treating cervical intraepithelial lesions by excising the affected part of the cervical epithelium using an electric wire loop. It affords the clinician to send the excised tissue for histopathology

3.6. Visual Inspection with Acetic acid (VIA)

VIA is based on the white appearance of dysplastic cervical epithelium after exposure to dilute 3-5% acetic acid (vinegar) for two to three minutes. The mechanism underlying the change is thought to be secondary to acetic acid's dehydrating effect on cellular cytoplasm and its ability to coagulate cellular proteins, the latter of which are usually in greater amounts in epithelium harboring CIN. The result is less transmission and greater reflection of incandescent light off the surface of epithelium containing CIN, recorded as a white appearance to the human eye.

4.0. HYPOTHESIS

4.1. Study hypothesis

Individual cryotherapy–ineligible acetowhite lesions of the cervix correlate well with histopathologic outcomes of high grade cervical intraepithelial neoplasia (CIN 2+).

4.2. Null hypothesis

There is no association between high grade cervical intraepithelial neoplasia (CIN 2+) and individual cryotherapy–ineligible acetowhite lesions of the cervix.

5.0. OBJECTIVES

5.1. Main Objective

To determine the association between high grade cervical intraepithelial neoplasia (CIN 2+) and individual acetowhite cryotherapy-ineligible lesion types, as determined by cervicography.

5.2. Specific Objectives

1. To determine the frequency of high grade cervical disease for individual cryotherapy-ineligible acetowhite lesions of the cervix

2. To establish the association between individual cryotherapy-ineligible acetowhite lesions of the cervix and high grade cervical disease

6. 0. METHODOLOGY

6.1. Study population

Women referred to the University Teaching Hospital gynecologic cancer prevention unit for histologic evaluation of cryotherapy-ineligible lesions were included in the study. Cryotherapy-ineligible lesions were defined as acetowhite lesions that do not meet criteria for cryotherapy. They include: acetowhite lesions that extend into endocervix beyond complete visualization; lesions occupying greater than 75% of the transformation zone; lesions with abnormal vessels (mosaicism, punctations or atypical vessels), thick lesions and satellite lesions. Females younger than 18 years and those with frankly invasive cervical cancer were excluded from the study. We also excluded women with more than one indication for histopathologic evaluation.

6.2. Study Design

A cross sectional observational study was designed. All women referred for histologic evaluation of cryotherapy-ineligible acetowhite lesions were asked to participate in the study after explaining the objectives. Consenting women were then asked to respond to a questionnaire asking for demographic and medical information. Participants also gave permission to use histopathologic results for their LEEP specimens. These specimens were collected as part of standard procedure in the management of cryotherapy-ineligible acetowhite lesions of the cervix. Histologic evaluation of LEEP specimens was done at the pathology laboratory of the University Teaching Hospital. Pathology results collected from the laboratory were recorded as: Normal histology, benign lesion, CIN 1, CIN 2, CIN 3, or micro-invasive cancer. Each result was further graded as either: High grade cervical disease ($\geq$ CIN 2), or Not High grade cervical disease (CIN 1 or less).

6.3. Sample size

A set of standard and comprehensive methods for reporting investigations of diagnostic tests known as STARDS (Standards for reporting diagnostic accuracy) was used to determine sample size. The STARD recommendations do not make specific recommendations for the number of participants. Despite the absence of specific recommendations for sample size calculation, 100 to 200 participants are usually adequate for tests in which the pretest probability is moderately high.[xli] In this study it was assumed that the prevalence of high grade cervical disease in the general population for the lesions under study and therefore the pretest probability was in the range of 50 percent. Consequently a sample size of 96 participants was calculated for the study (at 95% confidence interval and a maximum random error of 0.1 degrees of precision at estimated prevalence of 50%). To compensate for non-evaluable participants, 130 women were enrolled.

6.4. Ethical considerations

Before commencing enrolment, ethical approval was obtained from the University of Zambia Biomedical Research Ethics Committee. Eligible participants were enrolled in the study only after obtaining informed consent. Client confidentiality was maintained throughout the study. LEEP specimens were given unique identifier numbers before being sent to the laboratory. The identities of the participants were only known by core study staff directly involved in evaluating the clients. Members of the University of Zambia Biomedical Research Ethics Committee also have access to participant identity.

6.5. Outcome measures

The primary outcome measure of the study was the histologic diagnosis of high grade cervical disease for each specific cryotherapy-ineligible acetowhite lesion of the cervix. The secondary outcome measures included the frequency of specific cryotherapy-ineligible acetowhite lesions and the frequency of various histologic outcomes. The HIV serostatus of all participants was also recorded.

6.6. Statistical analysis

Collected data was imported to a statistical package for Social Scientists (SPSS Version 17.0) for widows and analyzed by a biostatistician. Descriptive and analytic evaluation was done. Descriptive analysis of baseline characteristics of the participants included mean & standard deviation for age, and then frequencies for marital status, educational level and monthly house hold income. The proportion of participants that was HIV positive was determined. Percentages of women with high grade cervical disease for each lesion under study were calculated. The association between high grade cervical disease and specific cryotherapy-ineligible lesions were determined using a logistic regression model. The confounding factors studied were: age, gravidity, parity, education status, average monthly household income, and HIV status.

7.0. RESULTS

A total of 130 women, each with a single cryotherapy -ineligible cervical lesion type, were enrolled into the study from April 2009 to October 2009.

Mean age of the participants was 33.5 years (range 19-55years) while the median age was 33. Fourteen (10.8%) of the 130 participants had never been married while 91 (70%) were married. 12 of the 130 participants (9.2%) were either divorced or separated and 13 (10%) were widowed. The education status of the study population was as follows: 15 of 130 (11.5%) had no formal education; 66 (50.8%) had some primary education; 40 (30.8%) had some secondary education; while 9 (6.9%) had some tertiary education. 89 of the 130 participants came from households that earned less than five hundred thousand Zambian Kwacha per month (K500, 000); while 41 (31.5%) were from households that earned at least K500, 000 per month (approximately $100) (see Table 1).

The average age at first sexual intercourse was 17. Forty-one of all participants (31.5%) had their first sexual intercourse before the age of 16 years; 71 (54.6%) were aged from 16 to 19 years while 18 (13.8%) were at least 20 years old at their first sexual intercourse (Table 2).

Six (4.6%) of the participants had not been pregnant before. The median gravidity was 3. The average number of pregnancies was 3.32, while the mode was 2 (see Table 3).

Nine (6.9%) of the participants were nulliparous. The median parity was three. 22 participants (16.9%) were grand multiparous (at least 5 parturitions).The average parity was 6 (see Table 4).

Table 1: Baseline characteristics of the sample population

Characteristic	Frequency	Percent
Grouped Age (in years		
<20	1	0.8
20-29	42	32.3
30-39	62	47.7
40+	25	19.2
Total	130	100
Marital status		
Never married	14	10.8
Married	91	70
Divorced/separated	12	9.2
Widowed	13	10
Total	130	100
Education level		
No formal education	15	11.5
Primary education	66	50.8
Secondary education	40	30.8
Tertiary education	9	6.9
Total	130	100
Estimated house hold income per month (in Zambian Kwacha)		
K500, 000 or less	89	68.5
More than K500, 000	41	31.5
Total	130	100

Table 2 :Age at first sexual intercourse

	Frequency
<16 years	41
16-19	71
20-25	18
All	130

Table 3 : Total number of pregnancies

	Frequency
No pregnancy	6
1-5 pregnancies	103
≥6 pregnancies	21
All	130

Table 4 :Parity

	Frequency
0	9
1-4	99
≥5	22
All	130

The HIV serostatus of the participants was as follows: 76 out of 130 (58.5%) were HIV positive; 28 (21.5%) were seronegative ; 26 participants (20%) did not know their status. Of the 76 HIV positive patients, 8 (10.5%) had been on HAART for less than 6 months. 23 (20.3%) had been on HAART for greater than 6 months. 45 (59.21%) were HAART naive (Tables 5 and 6).

The distribution of acetowhite lesions in the study sample was as follows: 48 of the 130 participants (36.9%) had acetowhite lesions occupying greater than 75% of the transformation zone; 35 (26.9%) had lesions disappearing into the cervical os beyond complete visualization; 20 (15.4%) had lesions too thick for cryotherapy. 13 participants had abnormal vessels: 6 (4.6%) had punctations; 5 (3.9%) had mosacism; and 2(1.5%) had atypical vessels. 14 participants had post treatment lesions: 11(8.5%) had post cryotherapy lesions and 3(2.3%) had post LEEP lesions (persistent lesion at least 6 months after treatment with cryotherapy or LEEP respectively).

Histopathologic outcomes for 27 (20.8%) of the participants was normal. 21 participants (16.2%) had benign lesions. Benign lesions were defined as histopathologic finding of cervicitis, polyp, cervical ulcer and schistosomiasis. 39 (30%) had CIN 1. 13 (10%) had CIN 2. 28 (21.5%) had CIN 3. Microinvasive cancer was diagnosed in 2 participants (1.54%). One participant with microinvasive cancer had a lesion occupying greater than 75 % of the transformation zone while the other had a lesion disappearing into the cervical os beyond complete visualization (Table 7).

The investigator defined high grade cervical disease to comprise participants with CIN2, CIN3 and microinvasive cancer. Low grade cervical disease was defined so as to include participants with benign lesions and CIN 1. Overall 43 participants (33.1%) had high grade cervical disease. 81 (66.9%) had either low grade cervical disease (46.2%) or normal histology (20.8%).

Table 8 shows the distribution of high grade cervical disease for various lesions: 26 (60.5%) women with high grade cervical disease had lesions occupying greater than 75% of the transformation zone while 22 (25.3%) women without high grade cervical disease also had lesions occupying greater than 75% of the transformation zone. 3 (7%) women with high grade cervical disease had lesions disappearing into the cervical os compared with 32 (36.8%) of women without high grade

Table 5 : HIV status of all participants	
	Frequency
Negative	28
Positive	76
Unknown	26
All	130

Table 6: Duration on HAART for the 76 HIV positive participants	
	Frequency
≤ 6 months	8
> 6months	23
Never taken antiretroviral drugs	45
All	76

Table 7: Frequency of specific histopathology results

Pathology result	Frequency
Normal histology	27
Benign lesions	21
CIN 1	39
CIN 2	13
CIN 3	28
Microinvasive	2
All	130

Table 8: Association between specific acetowhite lesions of the cervix and high grade cervical disease as dependent variable. Values expressed as odds ratios (OR) with corresponding 95% CI

Lesion Type	High grade cervical disease/ total	OR (95% CI)	Multivariable OR (95% CI)
Lesion >75% of Transformation zone			
No	17/82	Reference	
Yes	26/48	4.5 (2.1 – 9.9); P<0.001	2.2 (1.4 – 3.4), P=0.01.
Lesion extends into cervical os			
No	40/95	Reference	
Yes	3/35	0.1 (0.04 – 0. 45); P<0.001	
Lesion too thick for cryotherapy			
No	36/110	Reference	
Yes	7/20	1.1 (0.4 – 3.0); P=0.84	
Lesion with atypical vessels			
No	43/128	Reference	
Yes	0/2		
Lesion with punctations			
No	42/124	Reference	
Yes	1/6	0.4 (0.04 –3.45); P=0.38	
Lesion with mosaicism			
No	42/125	Reference	
Yes	1/5	0.5(0.1– 4.6); P=0.53	
Post-cryotherapy lesion			
No	40/119	Reference	
Yes	3/11	0.7 (0.2 – 2.9); P=0.67	
Post-LEEP Lesions			
No	41/127	Reference	
Yes	2/3	4.2 (0.4 – 47.6); P=0.21	

cervical disease. 7 (16.3%) of women with high grade cervical disease had lesions too thick for cryotherapy. 13 (14.9%) of women without high grade cervical disease had lesions too thick for cryotherapy.

Of the 6 women with punctations 1 (16.7%) had high grade cervical disease. Of the 5 women that had cervical lesions with mosaicism, 1 (20%) had high grade cervical disease on histology. To increase the evaluable size, participants with punctations and mosaicism were combined and analyzed as abnormal vessels. The percentage of lesions with abnormal vessels that were high grade cervical disease was calculated: 2 of the 13 participants with abnormal vessels (15.4%) had high grade cervical disease. Neither of the 2 women with atypical vessels on cervicography had high grade cervical disease on histopathology. Both of them were low grade cervical disease. Of the 11 post-cryotherapy lesions, 3 (27.3%) were high grade cervical disease. There was no statistically significant association found between post-LEEP lesions and high grade cervical disease. 2(4.7%) of women with high grade cervical disease had post-LEEP lesions compared with 1 (1.1%) of women without high grade cervical disease.

There was no association between age, parity, household income, or education status of the participants and high grade cervical disease. However there was an association between high grade cervical disease and HIV status. The odds of having high grade cervical disease were 5 fold higher for HIV sero-positive women with cryotherapy-ineligible lesions than for HIV sero-negative women with similar lesions.

Logistic regression was conducted for the study parameters that were associated with high grade cervical disease. After adjusting for age, gravidity, parity, education status, average monthly household income, and HIV status, the odds of having high grade cervical disease were 2.2 times higher for women with lesions occupying greater than 75% of transformation zone ,OR 2.2 (95% CI 1.4 – 3.4), p-value=0.01(Table 8).

8.0. DISCUSSION

In this study the incidence of negative and low grade histopathologic outcomes when cryotherapy-ineligible cervicography lesions were histologically evaluated was 66.9%. This finding arguably agrees with that of Bomfima et al (2005)[11] and Nuovo et al (1997).[10] Nuovo et al conducted a systemic review of the literature and found that the incidence of negative and low grade cervical disease when VIA positive lesions are histologically evaluated has been shown to range from 9.8 to 66.4% for high grade cervical lesion. Pfaendler et al (2005)[12] evaluated the histologic outcomes of cryotherapy-ineligible acetowhite lesions in general. That study found that 39.2% of acetowhite lesions were high grade cervical disease on histopathology. 60.8% of women diagnosed with cryotherapy-ineligible lesion on cervicography had negative or low grade cervical disease on histological examination.

This current study found an association between high grade cervical disease and acetowhite lesions occupying greater than 75% of the transformation zone. The odds of having high grade cervical disease were increased 2.2 times for women with acetowhite lesions occupying greater than 75% of the transformation zone, OR 2.2 (95% CI 1.4 – 3.4), p-value=0.01. This result renders support to the findings by Burghardt et al (1998)[37] who recommend that large or extensive

30

lesions involving more than three quadrants of the cervix should be investigated for possibilities of early invasive cancer. It may be assumed that the longer a cervical lesion persists, the more extensive it is likely to grow and subsequently the more likely that a dysplastic lesion may progress into a cancer.

In the current study, following logistic regression, there was no association between lesions disappearing into the cervical os beyond complete visualization (herein after called 'disappearing lesions') and high grade cervical disease. This finding was not completely unexpected. Although lesions disappearing into cervical os are regarded as cryotherapy-ineligible, the reason is not that they represent high grade cervical disease. LEEP is recommended for lesions disappearing into the cervical os because these lesions have been known to be resistant to cryotherapy.[38] The resistance to cryotherapy is explained by the fact that the full extent of lesions disappearing into the cervical os can not be ascertained and, therefore, cryonecrosis can not be guaranteed at the cranial limit of these lesions. This may result in failed cryotherapy and persistence of lesions. In the current study, however, despite the lack of association between disappearing lesions and high grade cervical disease, one of the only two cases of microinvasive carcinoma was a lesion disappearing into the cervical os. The other was a lesion occupying greater than 75% of the transformation zone.

In this study no statistically significant association was found between thick acetowhite lesions and high grade cervical disease. This finding is contrary to a long and widely held view with regard to thick acetowhite lesions of the cervix. Reid and Scalzi (1985)[39] have long held that "early preclinical cancer may appear as dense, thick chalky white areas with surface nodularity and irregularity, and with raised and rolled out margins. If cryotherapy is performed on such lesions, a biopsy must be taken before hand to exclude early cancer, otherwise LEEP is preferable." Although 35% of the 20 lesions that were too thick for cryotherapy had high grade cervical disease on histopathology, this figure was not statistically significant to justify an association between thick acetowhite cervical lesions and high grade cervical disease. Further studies, probably with a larger sample size may provide better data to refute or support this finding. However, the high percentage (35%) of thick lesions reported as high grade cervical disease seems to support the current practice of routinely conducting histopathologic evaluation for thick acetowhite lesions of the cervix.

In this study no association was found between abnormal vessels and high grade cervical disease. The investigator did not find any other studies that have specifically evaluated the histopathologic outcomes of cervical lesions with abnormal vessels. However, Reid and Scalzi (1985)[39] have reported that "as neoplastic process approaches the stage of invasive cancer, blood vessels can take on increasingly irregular bizarre patterns. Appearance of irregular vessels often indicates the first sign of invasion." Further studies are needed to specifically investigate the significance of abnormal vessels in the diagnosis of high grade cervical disease.

The current clinical practice is to undertake histologic evaluation of all acetowhite lesions that persist following treatment with either cryotherapy or LEEP. The persistence itself renders them refractory to treatment and therefore suspicious for cancer. In this study, no statistical association was found between post-cryotherapy lesions and high grade cervical disease. There was no independent data found in the literature search with which to compare this finding. However, the high percentage (27.3%) of post-cryotherapy lesions reported as high grade cervical disease would prompt many a clinician to consider histopathologic evaluation for all post-cryotherapy lesions. This study found no association between post-LEEP lesions and high grade cervical disease. This finding does not render support to the current clinical practice of histologically evaluating post-LEEP acetowhite lesions of the cervix.

9.0. CONCLUSIONS

Cryotherapy-ineligible acetowhite lesions occupying greater than 75% of the transformation zone diagnosed on cervicography are associated with histopathologic outcome of high grade cervical intraepithelial neoplasia.

10.0. STUDY LIMITATIONS

The investigator had initially planned to have one hired histopathologist to histologically evaluate the LEEP specimens, this was not possible and instead several pathologists were involved. Therefore, the histopathology data presented is subject to inter-rater bias. The sample size was small and this lowered the power of the study.

RECOMMENDATIONS

1. The current practice of referring women with cryotherapy-ineligible lesions for histologic evaluation should be done with more caution and may need to consider at least two provider assigned criteria for referral in order to reduce the incidence of negative histologic outcomes.

2. A larger study to evaluate specific histopathologic outcomes of cryotherapy-ineligible acetowhite lesions of the cervix will provide better results and is recommended.

11.0. APPENDICES

Appendix A - Information Sheet for Participants

Title Of Study: Histopathologic outcomes of women with cryotherapy-ineligible lesions on cervicography

Introduction

Dear Participant,

My name is.. I am asking you to participate in a research study to determine the true (histologic) diagnosis of white lesions found on the cervix on applying vinegar (acetic acid) to it. This study is being conducted by Dr. Samson Chisele. Dr Chisele is a postgraduate student at University of Zambia in the School of Medicine, department of Obstetrics and Gynaecology. The purpose of this study is to determine whether the current criteria used to refer women for histologic evaluation of acetowhite lesions of the cervix correlate well with histologic findings of high grade cervical disease. This information sheet gives you information about the study. If you understand and agree to take part in the study, you will be required to sign a consent form in the presence of a witness.

Explanation of Procedures

You will not be exposed to any experimental therapy in this study. All the following tests and measurements that will be made during the study are routine procedures to evaluate your cervical lesion. You would still need to undergo them even if you decided not to take part in the study.

Physical and Pelvic Examination: A routine general physical examination will be performed by a qualified medical doctor. This will be followed by a pelvic examination. To do this a speculum will be inserted in your vagina in order to expose and inspect your cervix. We will look for any sign of genital infection including sexually transmitted infection. Acetic acid will then be applied to your cervix using soaked cotton wool held in sponge holding forceps. The acetic acid will allow identification of any pre-cancerous lesions on the cervix which will appear white to the naked eye.

After 2 – 3 minutes of applying acetic acid to cervix, the doctor will again inspect the cervix to determine and describe the morphology of an acetowhite lesion. This description will be entered in a provided form. A picture of the cervix will be taken to show the lesion.

Performing Loop Electrosurgical Excision Procedure (LEEP): After determining morphology of lesion, the doctor will decide to take a sample of the lesion (punch biopsy) or remove the whole lesion using an electric current wire loop (LEEP). Before performing LEEP a local anaesthetic, lignocaine will be injected in four quadrants of the cervix in order to numb any pain.

Handling of specimens: The cervical specimen obtained will be stored in a container and sent for laboratory examination. You will then receive appropriate standard care depending on results of your specimen.

Alternative screening methods: Other methods of cervical cancer screening include Pap smear with colposcopy and HPV-DNA. These will not be offered to you. You will only be offered visual inspection of the cervix with acetic acid (VIA) and magnification of picture.

Risks and Discomforts: You will not encounter any additional risks or discomforts by virtue of your participation in the study. The above procedures are standard and are generally harmless. However, sometimes some minor complications can occur. These may be bleeding from cervix following biopsy. The bleeding, if it occurs, can quickly be stopped by the doctor. Some discomfort during the application of acetic acid to your cervix may occur although this will not last for more than a minute. You may also experience muscle cramps while LEEP is being performed but this will only last during the duration of the procedure. You will not be subjected to any experimental therapies.

Benefits: You may have no direct benefit from the study. However your participation in this study will provide valuable information to the medical community and the Cervical Cancer Prevention Programme in Zambia to ensure that LEEP is offered only to deserving clients and therefore reduce the cost and inconvenience associated with performing LEEP on women that may not need it.

Confidentiality: All information collected during the study will be kept in strict confidence. However core study staff and representatives of the biomedical research ethics committee of the University of Zambia will have access to your medical records, including your identity. Collected information including laboratory findings may be published for scientific purposes, but your personal identity will not be made public at any time.

Withdrawal without prejudice: You are free to withdraw from this study without prejudice of further care that you may enjoy at this institution.

Cost of participation: There will be no cost to you for participating in the study.

Payment for participation in study: You will not receive any payment for participating in this study.

Care for research related injuries: In this study, you will not be subjected to any new therapies. Therefore, you will not encounter any study related injuries. However, the investigator has made a provision for you to receive adequate care from the attending Consultant Gynaecologist within the clinic for any complications that may be encountered in standard practice, including bleeding from the cervix that may occur following biopsy.

Questions: If you have any questions or any research related injuries, you can contact Dr. Samson Chisele of University of Zambia/University Teaching Hospital, Department of Obstetrics and Gynaecology, at Cell no 095 555 4669. If you have questions regarding your rights as a participant in research, you can contact Dr. E. M. Nkandu, Chairperson of the University of Zambia Biomedical Research Ethics Committee (REC), University of Zambia, Ridgeway campus, P.O. Box 50110, Lusaka. Tel: 254641. Dr. Nkandu can be reached between 08:00hrs and 19:00hrs from Monday to Friday.

Appendix B - Informed consent

Title Of Study: Histopathologic outcomes of women with cryotherapy-ineligible lesions on cervicography

I have understood the purpose and procedures that will be involved in this study. I have willingly agreed to participate in the study and indicate this agreement by my signature below:

_____	_____	_____
Participant's name	Participant's signature/ Thumb print	Date

_____	_____	_____
Witness's name	Signature of Witness	Date

_____	_____	_____
Name of person obtaining consent	Signature of person obtaining consent	Date

Appendix C - Questionnaire

Title of Study: Histopathologic outcomes of women with cryotherapy-ineligible lesions on cervicography

1) Date of enrolment (DD/MM/YY)... / ... /...   2) Referring health facility:......

3) Reason for referral: Cryotherapy ineligible lesion=1   Failed cryotherapy=2

post LEEP=3   Other =4

4) CCIP # ....- ... /..... 5) UTH ID no........./ ...…   6) Study no: CIL ...

Personal Details

7) Patient's Last name................... Patient's First name...................

8) Age known   Yes=1   No=2   9) Date of birth (DD/MM/YY) .... / ../ ...

10) Age at last birth day (in years)...

(11) Household income/month (in Kwacha): <500,000=1   >500,000=2

12) Education level: No formal =1   Primary =2   Secondary =3   Tertiary=4

13) Marital status: Single=1   Married=2   Divorced/Separated=3   Widowed=4

14) Occupation:House wife=1   Formal sector=2   Informal sector=3
Other specify=4

Symptoms and Concerns

15) Vaginal/ vulval itching Yes=1   No=2   16) Vaginal discharge: Y=1
No=2

17) Pelvic or lower abdominal pain or tenderness: Yes=1 No=2   18) Fever:
Yes=1 No=2

19) Pain or burning with intercourse or urination: Yes=1
No=2

Obs/Gyn History

20) LMP (DD/MM/YY)   21) Menstrual blood flow: Heavy=1   Moderate=2
Scanty=3

22) Associated abdominal pain: Painful periods=1   No pain=2

23) Menstrual cycle regularity: Regular =1   Irregular=2

24) Age in years at first sexual Intercourse: ………….

25) Time of first sexual contact: Before onset of menses=1   After onset of
menses=2

26) History of bleeding during or after coitus   Yes =1   No=2

27) Total number of pregnancies…… 28) Number of abortions……………….

29) Current contraceptive use :(circle):   None=1   Natural method=2

Oral contraceptive pills=3 Injectable/implanted hormones=4

IUD=5   Condom/barrier methods=6   Tubal ligation=7

Hysterectomy=8

Past Medical History

30) Did you ever have a Pap smear test?   Yes=1   No=2

31) How long ago was your last Pap smear test? (in years) ……………

32) History of cervical cancer in any family member: Yes=1   No=2

33) Known HIV status: Y=1   N=2   34) Most recent HIV test: Positive=1
Negative=2

35) If positive, how long ago in months was test taken? ....

36) Any history of taking ARVs?   Yes=1   No=2

37) If on ARVs , how long have you taken them? ………………………..

Clinical Evaluation

38) General condition: Good=1   Fair=2   Poor=3

Visual inspection with acetic acid (VIA)

39) Lesion suspicious for cancer?   Yes =1   No=2

40) VIA done: Yes =1   No=2   41) VIA test results: positive=1   Negative=2

(If VIA positive, describe the morphology of the lesion)

42) Lesion extends into cervical os beyond complete visualization: Yes =1
No=2

43) Lesion Covers > 75%   of transformation zone: Yes =1   No=2

44) Atypical vessels: Yes=1   No=2   45) Punctations: Yes=1   No=2

46) Mosaicism: Yes=1   No=2   47) Too thick for Cryotherapy   Yes=1   No=2

48) Post cryotherapy Lesion: Yes=1 No=2   49) Post LEEP Lesion: Yes=1
No=2

Appendix D - Histopathology Report Form

CERVICOGRAPHY STUDY

UTH File No:………………..   CCPIZ#……….-…………./

……………....

Study No: CIL……………..   Date:

………………..

Brief history and examination:…………………………………………………

Diagnosis:………………………………………………………………………

Specimen:………………………………………………………………………

Examination required:

…………………………………………………………………………

Requesting Doctor……………………………..……   Signature:…….

……………………….

Histopathology Report

I. Gross Appearance: ………………………………………………………..

…………………………………………………………………………………

II. Microscopic Appearance:……………………………………..……………

……………………………………………………………………………………

……………………………………………………………..

………………………………………………….

……………………………………………………..………

Diagnosis :(report as: Normal, benign lesion, CIN 1, CIN 2, CIN 3, or

microinvasive cancer)

……………………….

……………………………………………………………………………………

Date of report: ……………………….

Name of pathologist: …………………………….   Signature:

……………………….

Grading of histopathology result to be done by principal investigator (report as

High grade cervical disease or Not high grade cervical disease)

…………………………………………………………………………………………

…………

12.0. REFERENCES

[i]   Cronje HS, Parham GP, Cooreman BF, et al. A comparison of four screening methods for cervical neoplasia in a developing country. *Am J Obstet Gynecol.* 2003;188:395-400.

[ii]   Mandelblatt JS, Lawrence WF, Gaffikin L, et al. Costs and benefits of different strategies to screen for cervical cancer in less developed countries. *J Natl Cancer Inst.*2002;94:1469-1483.

[iii]   Sankaranarayanan R, Basu P, Wesley RS, et al. Accuracy of visual screening for cervical neoplasia: results from an IARC multicentre study in India and Africa. *Int J Cancer.* 2004;110:907-913.

[iv]   Sankaranarayanan R, Esmy PO, Rajkumar R, et al. Effect of visual screening on cervical cancer incidence and mortality in Tamil Nadu, India: a cluster-randomised trial. *Lancet.* 2007;4(370):398-406.

[v]   Denny L, Kuhn L, De Souza M, Pollack AE, Dupree W, Wright TC Jr. Screen-and-treat approaches for cervical cancer prevention in low-resource settings: a randomized controlled trial. *JAMA.* 2005;294:2173-2181.

[vi]   J.W. Sellors JW, Sankaranarayanan R.Colposcopy and Treatment of Cervical Intraepithelial Neoplasia. A Beginner's Manual. Lyon 2003/4. English version ISBN 92 832 0412 3

[vii]   Ferris DG, Greenberg MD Reid's Colposcopic Index. J Fam Pract. 1994 Jul; 39(1): 6570.

[viii] Nuovo, J., Melnikov, J., Willan, A.R., & Chan, N.K. (2000) Treatment outcomes for squamous intraepithelial lesions. Int. J. Gynaecol. Obstet., 68, 25-33.

[ix]   Martin-Hirsch, P.L., Paraskevaidis, E., & Kitchener, H. (2000) Surgery for cervical intraepithelial neoplasia. Cochrane Database Syst. Rev., 2, CD001318.

[x]   Nuovo J, Melnikow J, Hutchison B, Paliescheskey M. Is cervicography a useful diagnostic test? A systematic overview of the literature. J Am Board Fam Pract. 1997 Nov-Dec;10(6):390-7

[xi]   Bomfima S, Santana-Francoa E, Bahamondesb L. Visual inspection with acetic acid for cervical cancer detection International Journal of Gynecology and Obstetrics (2005) 88, 65—66

[xii]   Pfaendler KS, Mwanahamuntu MH, Sahasrabuddhe VV, Mudenda V, Stringer JS, Parham GP. Management of cryotherapy-ineligible women in a "screen-and-treat" cervical cancer prevention program targeting HIV-infected women in Zambia: Lessons from the field. *Gynecol Oncol* 2008.

[xiii] WHO. *Preventing chronic diseases: a vital investment.* Geneva 2005.

[xiv]   Ferlay J, Bray F, Pisani P, Parkin DM. GLOBOCAN 2002 cancer incidence. Mortality and prevalence worldwide. IARC CancerBase No. 5 version 2.0. Lyon: IARC Press; 2004.

Bosch, F.X., Manos, M.M., Munoz, N., Sherman, M., Jansen, A.M., Peto, J., Schiffman, M.H., Moreno,V., Kurman, R., & Shah, K.V. (1995) The IBSCC Study Group. Prevalence of human papillomavirus in cervical cancer: a worlwide perspective. J. Natl. Cancer. Inst., 78, 796-802.

Walboomers, J.M.M., Jacobs, M.V., Manos, M.M., Bosch, F.X., Kummer, J.A., Shah, K.V., Snijders, P.J., Peto, J., Meijer, C.J., & Munoz, N. (1999) Human papillomavirus is a necessary cause of invasive cervical cancer worldwide. J. Pathol., 189, 12-19.

Thomas, G.M. (2000) Concurrent chemotherapy and radiation for locally advanced cervical cancer: the new standard of care. Semin. Radiat. Oncol., 10, 44-50

Franco, E.L., Rohan, T.E., & Villa, L.L. (1999) Epidemiologic evidence and human papillomavirus infection as a necessary cause of cervical cancer. J. Natl. Cancer Inst., 91, 506-511.

Tate DR, Anderson RJ. Recrudescence of cervical dysplasia among women who are infected with the human immunodeficiency virus: a case-control analysis. Am J Obstet Gynecol 2002; 186: 880-2.

Ho GY, Bierman R, Beardsley L, Chang CJ, Burk RD. Natural history of cervicovaginal papillomavirus infection in young women. NEJM 1998; 338:423-428.

Heard I, Tassie JM, Schmitz V, Mandeelbrot l, Katatchkiine MD, Orth G.Increased risk of cervical disease among human immunodeficiency virus-infected women with severe immunosuppression and high human papillomavirus load. Obstet Gynecol 2000;96:403-09.

Duerr A, Kicke B, Warren D, Shah K, Burk R, Peipert JF, et al. Human papillomavirus-associated cervical cytologic abnormalities among women with or at risk of infection with human immunodeficiency virus. Am J Obstet Gynecol 200; 184: 584-90.

Delmas MC, Larsen C, van Benthem B, Hmaers FF, Bergeron C, Poveda JD, et al. Cervical squamous intraepithelial lesions in HIV-infected women: prevalence, incidence and regression. European Study Group on the Natural History of HIV Infection in Women. AIUDS 2000;14:1775-84.

Volkow P, Rubi S, Lizano M, Carillo A, Vilar-Compte D, Garcia-Carranca A, et al. High prevalence of oncogenic human papillomavirus in the genital tract of women with human immunodeficiency virus. Gynecol Oncol 2001;82:27-311.

Conti M, Agarossi A, Parazzini F, Muggiasca ML, Boschuni A, Negri E, et al. HPV, HIV infection and risk of cervical intraepithelial neoplasia in former intravenous drug abusers. Gynecol Oncol 1993;49:344-8.

Palefsky JM, Minkoff H, Kalish LA, Levine A, Sacks HS, Garcia P, et al. Cervicovaginal human papillomavirus infection in human immunodeficiency virus-1. (HIV) - positive and high-risk HIV-negative women. J Natl Cancer Inst 1999; 91: 226-36.

Conley LJ, Ellerbrock TV, Bush TJ, Chiasson MA, Sawo D, Wright TC. HIV-1 infection and risk of vulvovaginal and perianal condylomata acuminate and intraepithelial neoplasia: a prospective cohort study. Lancet 2002; 359: 108-13.

^{xxviii}

    Ferris DG, Payne P, Frisch LE, Milner FH, diPaola FM, Petry LJ. Cervicography: adjunctive cervical cancer screening by primary care clinicians. J Fam Pract. 1993 Aug;37(2):158-64.

^{xxix}

    Cecchini S, Bonardi R, Mazzotta A, Grazzini G, Iossa A, Ciatto S. Testing cervicography and cervicoscopy as screening tests for cervical cancer. Tumori. 1993 Feb 28;79(1):22-5

^{xxx}

    Frisch LE, Milner FH, Ferris DG. Naked-eye inspection of the cervix after acetic acid application may improve the predictive value of negative cytologic screening. J Fam Pract. 1994 Nov;39(5):457-60

^{xxxi}

    Denny L, Kuhn L, Pollack A, Wright Jr TC. Direct visual inspection for cervical cancer screening: an analysis of factors influencing test performance. Cancer 2002 Mar 15;94(6):1699–707.

^{xxxii}

    Baldauf JJ, Dreyfus M, Ritter J, Meyer P, Philippe E. Cervicography. Does it improve cervical cancer screening? Acta Cytol. 1997 Mar-Apr;41(2):295-301

^{xxxiii}

    Numnum TM, Kirby TO, Leath CA 3rd, Huh WK, Alvarez RD, Straughn JM Jr. A prospective evaluation of "see and treat" in women with HSIL Pap smear results: is this an appropriate strategy? J Low Genit Tract Dis. 2005 Jan;9(1):2-6

^{xxxiv}

    Szurkus DC, Harrison TA. Loop excision for high-grade squamous intraepithelial lesion on cytology: correlation with colposcopic and histologic findings. Am J Obstet Gynecol. 2003 May;188(5):1180-2

^{xxxv}

    Charoenkwan K, Srisomboon J, Suprasert P, Siriaunkgul S, Khunamornpong S. Histopathological outcomes of women with squamous cell carcinoma on cervical cytology. Asian Pac J Cancer Prev. 2006 Jul-Sep;7(3):403-6.

^{xxxvi}

    Howells RE, O'Mahony F, Tucker H, Millinship J, Jones PW, Redman CW. How can the incidence of negative specimens resulting from large loop excision of the cervical transformation zone (LLETZ) be reduced? An analysis of negative LLETZ specimens and development of a predictive model. BJOG. 2000 Sep;107(9):1075-82.

^{xxxvii}

    Burghardt, E., Pickel, H., & Girardi, F. (1998) Colposcopy Cervical Pathology. Textbook and Atlas. Thieme, New York.
^{xxxviii}

    Coppleson, M., Dalrymple, J.C., & Atkinson, K.H. (1993b) Colposcopic differentiation of abnormalities arising in the transformation zone. In Wright, V.C. (Ed). Contemporary Colposcopy. Philadelphia: WB Saunders.
^{xxxix}

    Reid, R., & Scalzi, P. (1985) Genital warts and cervical cancerVII. An improved colposcopic index for differentiating benign papillomaviral infections from high-grade cervical intraepithelial neoplasia. Am. J. Obstet. Gynecol., 153, 611-618
^{xl}

Coppleson, M., Reid, B., & Pixley, E. (1986) Colposcopy, 3rd Edition, Charles C Thomas, Springfield.
xli

Richard KR. Studying a study and testing a test-How to read the manual evidence. 5th edition,2005. Lippincott Williams and Wilkins.

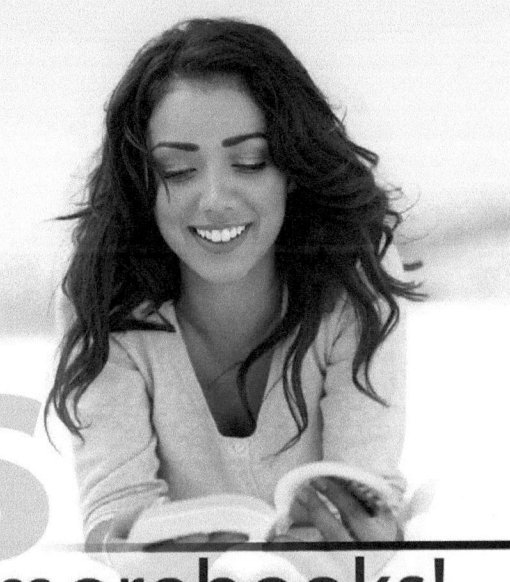
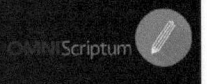

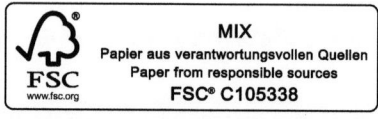

Printed by Books on Demand GmbH, Norderstedt / Germany